RESEARCH PRESENTATIONS OF DIETETIC INTERNSHIP PARTICIPANTS

SUMMARY SERIES No. 1   **APRIL 2010**

RESEARCH PROCEEDINGS - NUTRITION AND FOOD SECTION

CHERYL L. ATKINSON

Associate Professor and
Director, Dietetic Internship Program

SOUTHERN UNIVERSITY AND A&M COLLEGE
College of Agricultural Family and Consumer Sciences
Division of Family and Consumer Sciences

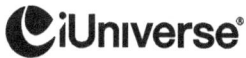

Research Presentations of Dietetic Internship Participants
Research Proceedings - Nutrition and Food Section

iUniverse books may be ordered through booksellers or by contacting:

iUniverse
1663 Liberty Drive
Bloomington, IN 47403
www.iuniverse.com
1-800-Authors (1-800-288-4677)

Because of the dynamic nature of the Internet, any web addresses or links contained in this book may have changed since publication and may no longer be valid. The views expressed in this work are solely those of the author and do not necessarily reflect the views of the publisher, and the publisher hereby disclaims any responsibility for them.

Any people depicted in stock imagery provided by Thinkstock are models, and such images are being used for illustrative purposes only. Certain stock imagery © Thinkstock.

ISBN: 978-1-4917-4902-9 (sc)
ISBN: 978-1-4917-4903-6 (e)

Printed in the United States of America.

iUniverse rev. date: 11/07/2014

FOREWORD

The importance of student-conducted research cannot be over-stated.
Increased learning occurs when students are involved in original and on-going research at all levels of the process. When students are allowed the opportunity to integrate concepts learned in the didactic setting to real life situations, they have an ability to gain a better understanding of the subject matter being investigated.

The research presentations of the Southern University Dietetic Interns presented in this Research Proceeding, is the first in a series of original works designed and conducted by post-baccalaureate students enrolled in the supervised practice experience program known as the Dietetic Internship. This Graduate level program is housed in the College of Agricultural, Family and Consumer Sciences, in the Division of Family and Consumer Sciences and is in the Department of Human Nutrition and Food.

These first three papers, which comprise the first in this series, have established the tone and the level of quality that all other papers will achieve in the coming series.

The first paper is entitled: *Investigating the Relationship between Health Awareness Activities and Body Mass Index among 18-25 year olds in Baton Rouge, Louisiana.* (C. Lemoine and A. Weston)

The second paper is entitled: *Attitudes on Breastfeeding of a Select Group of Mothers and Comparison to Healthy People 2010 Goals.* (J. Lang and A. Heard)

The third paper is entitled: *Artificially Sweetened Beverage Consumption and Portion Control by African American Female College Students.* (C. Abels and D. Kenda)

These original research papers were submitted and presented at the Louisiana Dietetic Association's Annual Food and Nutrition Conference in 2010.

Special thanks to all members of the peer-review committee, whose insight, recommendations and support for this project were invaluable.

PEER-REVIEW COMMITTEE:

Verra Bachireddy PhD
Andra Johnson PhD
Calvin Walker PhD
Ivis Forrester PhD, RD

Editor:
Cheryl L. Atkinson PhD, RD, LDN

Staff:
Debbie Johnson Gwinn BS

INVESTIGATING THE RELATIONSHIP BETWEEN HEALTH AWARENESS ACTIVITIES AND BODY MASS INDEX AMONG 18-25 YEAR OLDS IN BATON ROUGE, LA

By:

Charlotte Lemoine, BS
Ashley Weston, BS

A research manuscript in Partial Fulfillment
Of the Requirements for the Southern University
Dietetic Internship Program

FOOD AND HUMAN NUTRITION
DIVISION OF FAMILY AND CONSUMER SCIENCES
COLLEGE OF AGRICULTURAL, FAMILY AND CONSUMER SCIENCES
SOUTHERN UNIVERSITY AND A&M COLLEGE

ABSTRACT

Objective: The purpose of this study is to compare health awareness media viewing and health class attendance, to body mass index (BMI) among young adults, aged 18-25, in Baton Rouge, LA.

Method: A survey consisting of questions about exposure to health media, health awareness classes attended and BMI was given to a total of 80 males and females aged 18-25, in the Baton Rouge Areal via email.

Statistical Analysis: Descriptive statistics were performed to compare the frequency of nutrition media and health classes on body mass index and eating habits.

Results: 70% of the participants surveyed, reported seeing three or more health promotion ads/month. 50% of those have a normal BMI and 45% are overweight or greater. 53% of the individuals have had only one health education class and of those 45% had a normal BMI and 53% were overweight or greater. Of the individuals with a normal BMI, 45% have had one nutrition class, and 71% see three or more nutrition ads a month. Also, among the individuals with a normal BMI, only 40% claim they eat balanced meals, 5% eat the recommended 4-5 servings of fruits and vegetables daily, 57% eat 1-2 servings of fruits and vegetables daily, 57% think of eating better daily, 24% actually attempt to eat better daily, and 38% buy healthier foods at the grocery store instead of convenience foods or eating out.

Conclusions: 70% of the participants see three or more ads a month and 54% of those participants have a normal BMI. These findings suggest that individuals who are reminded of health benefits may attempt to eat better more frequently and have a better BMI. Even though these individuals exhibited a normal BMI, the data suggests that their eating habits are unhealthy. Nutrition media appears to be more effective in improving knowledge but not poor eating habits. A likely reason why they have a normal BMI could be because of their activity level and not their eating habits. Perhaps a longitudinal study would give more comprehensible results. Health promotions media and classes could increase health awareness.

INTRODUCTION

Obesity is becoming a huge epidemic in America with 35 of women and 33 of men being obese based on the most recent NHANES survey. Based on the Behavioral Risk Factor Surveillance System, 19.1 of men and women ages 18-29 are obese.

Today young adults are faced with a fast paced, intense lifestyle with mounting work and school obligations. This leaves less time for meal planning, grocery shopping, and physical activity. In addition, Western culture uses food to socialize so choices are made rapidly without thought. Convenience foods are also readily available and are high in saturated fats and refined sugars.

Healthy People 2010 recommend five to nine servings of fruits and vegetables a day and based on many studies, the average American does not meet that recommended intake. Fruits and Vegetables are recommended to prevent chronic diseases such as heart disease, diabetes, and cancer. Overweight and Obesity is also associated with these chronic diseases. With this Knowledge, are we making healthier food choices?

The purpose of this research project was to find out if health classes and nutrition awareness media improves the knowledge and motivation to make healthier food choices and decrease body mass index.

OBJECTIVE

The purpose of this study is to compare health awareness media viewing and health classes attendance, to body mass index (BMI) among young adults, aged 18-25, in Baton Rouge, LA.

METHODS

Subjects included a convenience sample of 80 males and females ages 18-25, informally emailed with attachment of consent form and survey by the researchers. After signing a statement of informed consent, the subjects completed a 10 item type written survey. The survey instrument collected demographic and subjective information including sex, weight status, eating and shopping habits, and health awareness. Self-reported height and weight also were used to determine body mass index (BMI) and BMI categories. Data were analyzed using the Excel Data Analysis.

We compared Body Mass Index with the following:

- Fruit and vegetable intake
- Nutrition classes
- Promotional health ads

- Thoughts on eating better
- Attempts to eat better
- Grocery shopping habits
- Meal eating habits

RESULTS

A total of 80 participants completed the survey (56 female and 24 male.) of the participants surveyed, 70% reported seeing three or more health promotion ads/months. Of those, 50% have a normal BMI and 45% are overweight or greater. 53% of the individuals have had only one health education class and of those 45% had a normal BMI and 53% were overweight or greater. Of the individuals with a normal BMI, 45% have had one nutrition class, and 71% see three or more nutrition ads a month. Furthermore, among the normal weight individuals, 90% considered themselves a healthy weight. 50% of the obese group considered themselves a healthy weight. 65% of the overweight group considered themselves a healthy weight. Also, among the individuals with a normal BMI, only 40% claim they eat balanced meals, 5% eat 4-5 servings of fruits and vegetables daily, 57% eat 1-2 servings, 57% think of eating better daily, 24% actually attempt to eat better daily, and 38% buy healthier foods at the grocery store instead of convenience foods or eating out.

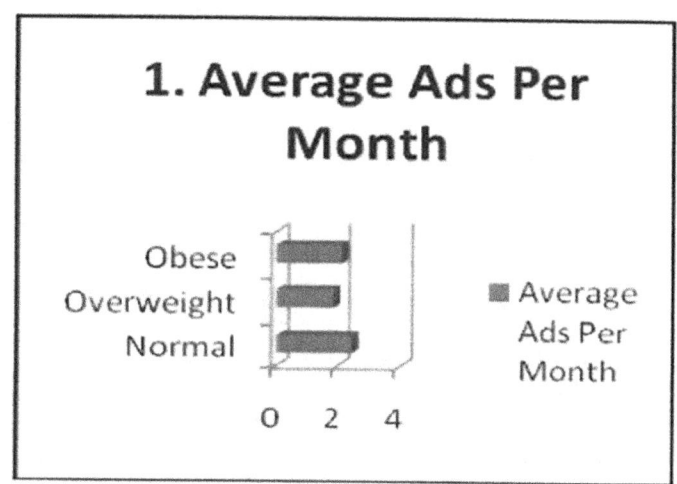

Table 1: Shows the average ads seen per month by participants whose BMI is obese, overweight, and normal.

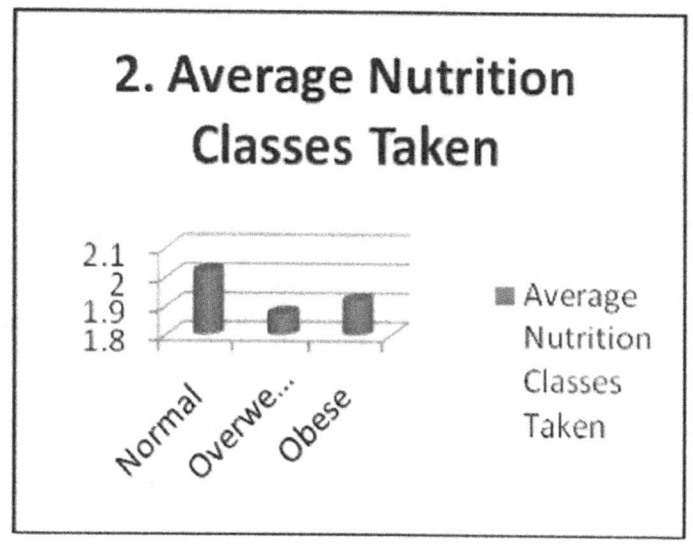

Table 2: Shows the average nutrition classes taken by participants whose BMI is normal, overweight, obese.

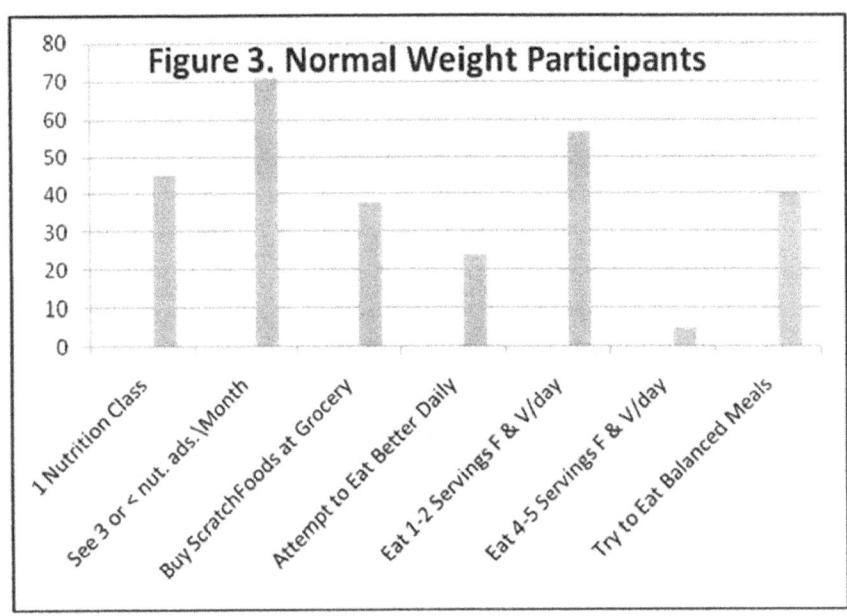

Table 3: Shows the number of participants whose BMI is normal who has seen at least one nutrition class, seen 3 or more ads per month, cooks their own food/buy scratch foods, attempt to eat better daily, eat 1-2 servings of fruits and vegetables daily, eats 4-5 servings of fruit and vegetables daily, and tries to eat balanced meals.

CONCLUSION AND DISCUSSION

Of the participants, 70% see three or more ads a month, 54% of those participants have a normal BMI. These findings suggest that individuals who are reminded of health benefits may attempt to eat better more frequently and have a better BMI. Even though these individuals exhibited a normal BMI, the data suggest their eating habits are unhealthy. Nutrition media appears to be more effective in improving knowledge but not poor eating habits. A likely reason why they have a normal BMI could be because of their activity level and not their eating habits. Perhaps a longitudinal study would give more comprehensible results. Health promotions media and classes could increase health awareness and the knowledge one has of nutrition but is only somewhat effective in changing an individuals eating habits. Furthermore, most overweight or obese individuals in this study considered themselves to be a healthy weight. If they were aware of their weight status, could that make them try harder to lower their BMI? This could be another study in itself.

APPENDIX A

(STUDY/PROJECT INFORMATION FOR HMAN SUBJECTS COMMITTEE)

STUDY/PROJECT INFORMATION FOR HUMAN SUBJECTS COMMITTEE

> Describe your study/project in detail for the Human Subjects Committee. Please include the following information.

TITLE: Health Awareness Among Young Adults

PROJECT DIRECTOR(S): Charlotte Lemoine, BS, Ashley Weston, BS (Dietetic Inter=FCSC 501 and 502), Cheryl Atkinson, PhD., RD, LDN (Professor, Human Nutrition and Food

EMAIL: Cheryl_atkinson@subr.edu

PHONE: 225-771-4660

DEPARTMENTS(S): Division of Family and Consumer Sciences, Human Nutrition and Food Program

PURPOSE OF STUDY/PROJECT: The purpose of the study is to measure the effects of health awareness on body mass index (BMI) and eating behavior among men and women, aged 18-25, in Baton Rouge, LA.

SUBJECTS: The subjects will be a convenience sample of approximately 100 young adults. We will informally approach the participants via email.

PROCEDURE: The subjects will be first asked to sign a Human Consent Form and then fill a 10 question survey that will take approximately 5 minutes.

INSTRUMENTS AND MEASURES TO INSURE PROTECTION OF CONFIDENTIALITY, ANONYMITY: The ten question survey titled health Awareness Among Young Adults developed by the researchers will be used to compare body mass index (BMI) and eating behavior in connection with health awareness. All collected information will be held confidential and only viewed by the researchers.

RISKS/ALTERNATIVE TREATMENTS: There are no risks or alternative treatments and participation is voluntary.

BENEFITS/COMPENSATION: There will be a drawing at the end of the study for a $10 gift card to Smoothie King.

SAFEGUARDS OF PHYSICAL AND EMOTIONAL WELL-BEING: This study involves no treatment. All information collected from the survey will be held strictly confidential. No one will be allowed access to the survey other than the residence.

> **Note:** Use the Human Subjects Consent form to briefly summarize information about the Study/project to participant and obtain their permission to participate.

APPENDIX B

(HUMAN SUBJECTS CONSENT FORM)

APPENDIX B

HUMAN SUBJECTS CONSENT FORM

> The following is a brief summary of the project in which you are asked to participate. Please read this information before signing the statement below.

TITLE: The effect of health awareness on BMI and eating behavior among men and women, aged 18-25, in Baton Rouge, LA.

PURPOSE OF STUDY/PROJECT: The purpose of this study is to measure the effects of health awareness on body mass index (BMI) and eating behavior among men and women, aged 18-25, in Baton Rouge, LA.

PROCEDURE: After signing this form, you will be asked to complete a 10-item survey that will take approximately 5 minutes. If you choose to do so, you will be entered into a drawing for a $10 gift card to Smoothie King.

INSTRUMENTS: A short confidential 10 question survey that will collect information about your gender, body mass index (BMI) and lifestyle approaches.

RISKS/ALTERNATIVE TREATMENTS: There are no risks or alternative treatments.

BENEFITS/COMPENSATION: You will be entered into a drawing for one $10 gift card to Smoothie King.

I, _____, attest with my signature that I have <u>read and understood the following description of the study</u>. "Health Awareness Among Young Adults", and its purpose and methods. I understand that my participation in this research is strictly voluntary <u>and my prescription or refusal to participate in this study will affect me in any way</u>. Further, I understand that I may withdraw at any time or refuse to answer any questions without penalty. Upon completion of the study, I understand that the results or my survey will be <u>confidential, accessible only to the principal investigators, myself, or a legally appointed representative</u>. I have not been requested to waive nor do I waive any of my rights related to participating in this study.

_____   _____

Signature of Participant   Date

CONTACT INFORMATION: The principal experimenters listed below may be reached to answer questions about the research, subjects' rights or related matters.

Charlotte Lemoine chemol8@gmail.com and Ashley Weston atw008@gmail.com

APPENDIX C

(SURVEY)

HEALTH AWARENESS AMONG YOUNG ADULTS

Instructions: Circle the answer that best describes you. Fill in the blanks.

1. Do you consider yourself a health weight?
   a. **YES**
   b. **NO**
2. Are you
   a. **Male**
   b. **Female**
3. Do this equation with your weight (in pounds) and height (in inches) and circle the range for your answer:
   Weight/height/height x 703=
   Ex: 130/65/65x703=21.6
   a. **18.4 or >**
   b. **18.5-24.9**
   c. **25-29.9**
   d. **30-34.9**
   e. **35-39.9**
   f. **40 or <**
4. How often do you see ads promoting nutritional health?
   a. **1x/month**
   b. **2x/month**
   c. **3x/month**
   d. **Hardly ever**
5. Have you ever taken a class on Nutritional health? (even in grade school or high school)
   a. **Once**
   b. **Twice**
   c. **Three times**
   d. **More**
6. How often do you THINK about eating better?
   a. **Daily**
   b. **Weekly**
   c. **Monthly**
   d. **Yearly**
   e. **Once in a few years**
   f. **Never**
7. How often do you actually make advances to eating better?
   a. **Daily**
   b. **Weekly**
   c. **Monthly**
   d. **Yearly**
   e. **Once in a few years**
   f. **Never**

8. How many ½ cup servings of fruits or vegetables do you eat on a daily basis?
   a. **0**
   b. **1-2**
   c. **2-3**
   d. **3-4**
   e. **4-5**
9. When you grocery shop, do you mostly buy:
   a. **Ingredients to cook food from scratch (fresh vegetables, raw meats, pasta or rice, fresh fruits, etc)**
   b. **Convenience foods (prepackaged foods on the shelves or in the freezer that are lower in price and easy to prepare)**
   c. **I don't grocery shop, I eat out mostly.**
10. When you prepare your plate, do you try to make the meal balanced (1 serving starch, 1 serving meat, 2 servings fruits or vegetables)
    a. **Always**
    b. **Half the time**
    c. **A third of the time**
    d. **Never**

ATTITUDES ON BREASTFEEDING OF A SELECT GROUP OF MOTHERS AND COMPARISON TO HEALTHY PEOPLE 2010 GOALS

By:

Judy Hand Lang BS
&
Arlene Heard BS

A research manuscript in Partial fulfillment of the Requirements of the Southern University Dietetic Internship

FOOD AND HUMAN NUTRITION
DIVISION OF FAMILY AND CONSUMER SCIENCES
COLLEGE OF AGRICULTURAL, FAMILY AND CONSUMER SCIENCES
SOUTHERN UNIVERSITY AND A&M COLLEGE

INTRODUCTION

Breast milk is the "gold standard" that infant formulas are measured against. Experts agree that the best milk for a human infant is mother's milk, more specifically, that infant's mother's milk. The Office of Surgeon General of the United States has made the following recommendations concerning breastfeeding. "Improve professional education in human lactation and breastfeeding; develop public education and promotional efforts; strengthen the support for breastfeeding; develop public education and promotional efforts; strengthen the support for breastfeeding in the health care system; develop a broad range of support services in the community; initiate a national breastfeeding promotion effort directed to women in the world of work; and expand research on human lactation and breastfeeding (U.S. Department of Health and Human Services, 2000). "One of the objectives of Healthy People 2010 is to increase the proportion of mothers who breastfeed their babies in the early postpartum period to 75% from a baseline of 64% in 1998, at 6 months to 50% from a baseline of 29% in 1998, at 1 year to 25% from a baseline of 16% in 1998 (Healthy People 2010, 2000).

The U. S. Preventive Services Task Force recommends structured breastfeeding education and behavioral counseling sessions to promote breastfeeding and found that these methods are associated with increased rates of initiation and continuation of breastfeeding for at least 3 months (U.S. Preventive Services Task Fore, 2008). LaLeche League International (LLI) is an organization that offers mother-to-mother support, encouragement, information, and education, and is an example of the type of counseling sessions that are available for a new mother (LaLeche League International, 2008).

The Centers for Disease Control and Prevention (CDC) report that by 3 months after birth, only 73.8% of women in the U.S. who are physically capable of breastfeeding attempt to do so. By 3 months after birth, only 30.5% do so, and by 6 months after birth, only 11.3% breastfed exclusively (CDC, 2008).

Factors that influence breastfeeding decisions as summarized in the U.S. Department of Health and Human Services (USDHHS) Blueprint for Action on Breastfeeding, are maternity care practices, interactions with health-care professionals, and workplace (U.S. Department of Health and Human Services, 2000). When work places provide support systems from supervisors, co-workers, and spouses, it helps to reduce work-family conflict and makes combining employment and breastfeeding more successful. (Morse and Bottorff, 1989).

The aims of this study were to investigate the reasons why women did not breastfeed their babies; what education they had received about breastfeeding; what support they had received when breastfeeding, if they chose to do so; what obstacles had to be overcome to breastfeed; and how the local, current generation of mothers in the area of Baton Rouge, LA are compared to the statistics of the United States on a national level. Another aim of this study was to find out if the local population of mothers had differences in the attitudes or experiences that reflected the mother's age range or ethnicity.

A survey was designed and distributed to the mothers at a daycare center in Baton Rouge, LA. The first page of the survey dealt with demographic data and questions as to why mothers chose not to breastfeed. If they had breastfed their babies, page two asked questions about the preparation they had received to breastfeed, the type of help received and if the help was useful, how long they breastfeed, and the reason(s) they ceased breastfeeding.

MATERIALS AND METHODS

A survey (see Appendix A) form was used to obtain information from mothers of children ages 0 to 3 years old. The survey was done in December 2008, at Parkview Baptist Preschool. A total of 75 surveys were distributed and 50 mothers participated in the survey. The subjects received a letter explaining who was conducting the study and for what it would be used. In order to facilitate more participation at a busy time of year, the survey was kept brief. If the mother had not breastfed her baby, only one page needed to be filled out. Permission from the director of the daycare was obtained. Teachers in the facility handed out the surveys to the mothers, who turned them back in to the teachers when completed.

The data were analyzed according to race, marital status, education level, employment status, type of breastfeeding preparation, how long after birth breastfeeding help was given, who gave breastfeeding help, what determined when the baby was fed, any supplemental feedings given to the baby, whether any pain was experienced initially in breastfeeding, the degree that the help obtained seemed to improve the situation, how long breast milk was given to the baby, and reasons given for not breastfeeding and for ceasing to breastfed.

The subject's ages ranged between 19-38 years. Directions to fill out the survey were for mothers to consider only their last child when answering the questions.

RESULTS

The sample of this study (n=49) includes White (n=42), Black (n=5), Asian (n=1) and Mexican (n=1) (Figure, 1) and the average age was 29.8 years. Compared to the population of Louisiana census 2000 (56.3% White, 40.0% Black, 2.6% others), our sample had 84% White, 10.2% Black, and 4.1% others. 93.6% of the breastfeeding mothers and 33.4% of the non-breastfeeding mothers had an education level of bachelor's degree or higher (Figure 2).

RESULTS

The sample of this study (n=49) includes White (n=42), Black (n=5), Asian (n=1) and Mexican (n=1) (Figure.1) and the average age was 29.8 years. Compared to the population of Louisiana Census 2000 (56.3% White, 40.0% Black, 2.6% others), our sample had 84% White, 10.2% Black, and 4.1% others. 93.6% of the breastfeeding mothers and 33.4% of the non-breastfeeding mothers had an education level of bachelor's degree or higher (Figure 2).

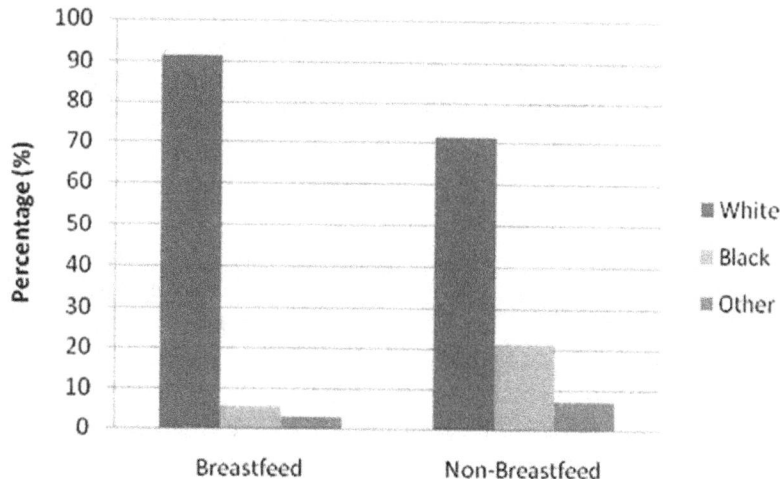

Figure 1. Race of the sample of this study (n=49).

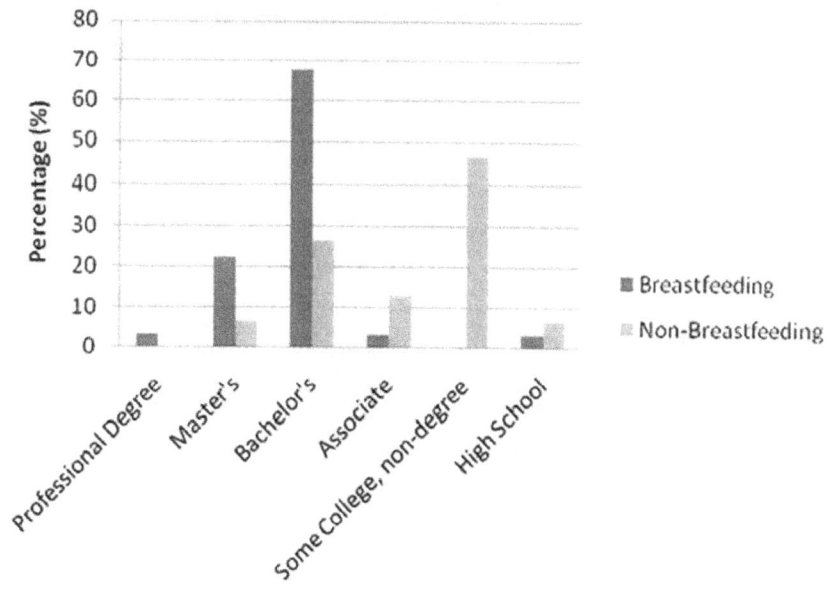

Figure 2. Education level of the participants.

Among the participants, 71.4% (n=35) of them had breastfed at some point and 28.6% (n=14) did not breastfed before. 55.6% of the respondents who had breastfed at some point had attended a class on breastfeeding, while only 6.8% of the non-breastfeeding mothers had attended a class on breastfeeding (Figure 3). The top three most important reasons for not breastfeeding were "Thought that formula is as good or better than breast milk", "Inconvenience", and "Had to go back to work or school" (Figure 4). 46.2% of the breastfeeding mothers fed their baby with water, formula or sugar water while they were in the hospital or birth center. Among the breastfeeding mothers, 11.1% (n=4) breastfed or gave pumped breast milk to the baby for at least 6 months after delivery, and 5.6% (n=2) breastfed for more than 12 months (Figure 5). The three main reasons for the stopping of breastfeeding for those who did stop were "Return to work/school or daycare", "Felt baby was old enough" and "Low milk supply" (Figure 6).

Among the participants, 71.4% (n=35) of them had breastfed at some point and 28.6% (n=14) did not breastfeed before. 55.6% of the respondents who had breastfed at some point had attended a class on breastfeeding, while only 6.8% of the non-breastfeeding mothers had attended a class on breastfeeding (Figure 3). The top three most important reasons for not breastfeeding were "Thought that formula is as good or better than breast milk", "Inconvenience", and "Had to go back to work or school" (Figure 4). 46.2% of the breastfeeding mothers fed their baby with water, formula or sugar water while they were in the hospital or birth center. Among the breastfeeding mothers, 11.1% (n=4) breastfed or gave pumped breast milk to the baby for at least 6 months after delivery, and 5.6% (n=2) breastfed for more than 12 months (Figure 5). The three main reasons for the stopping of breastfeeding for those who did stop were "Return to work/school or daycare", "Felt baby was old enough" and "Low milk supply" (Figure 6).

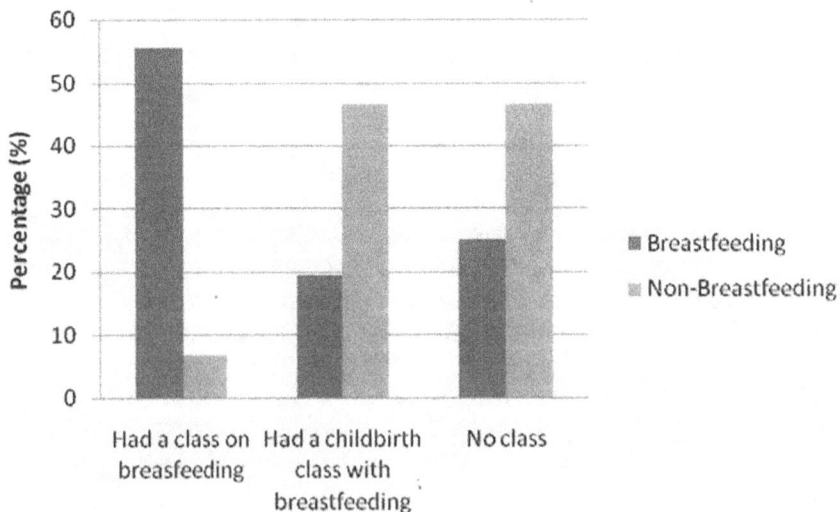

Figure 3. Percentage of participants who attended a class on breastfeeding, had a childbirth class with breastfeeding or did not have a breastfeeding class.

Figure 4. Reasons for not breastfeeding

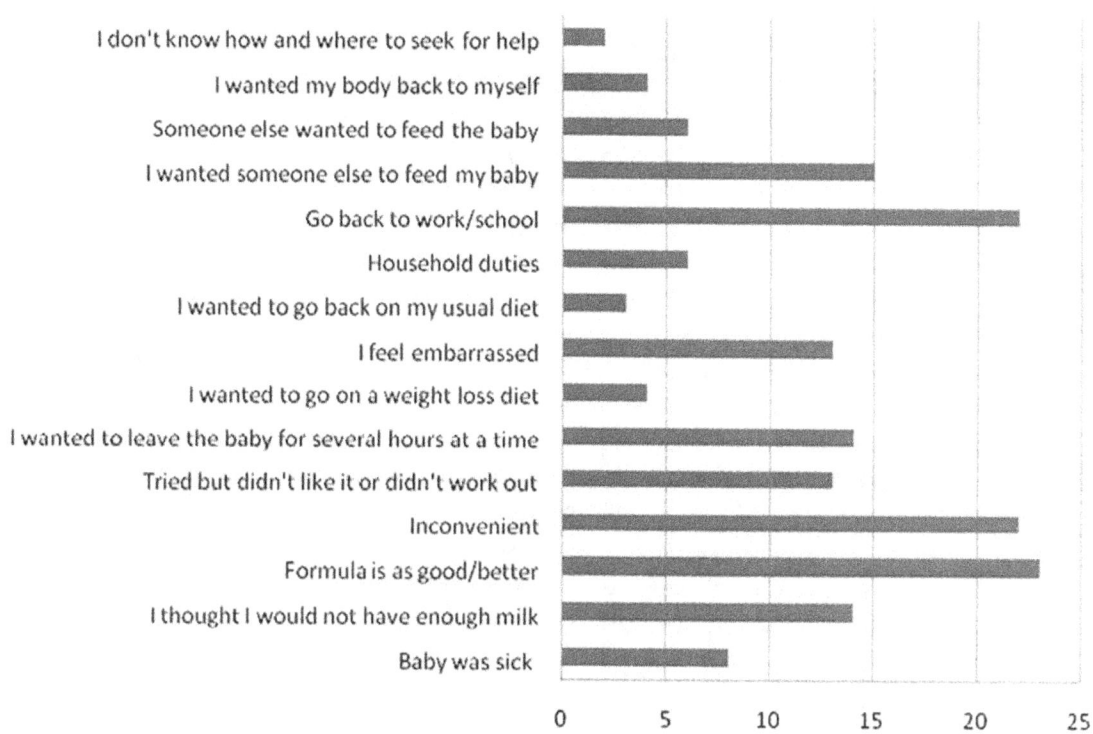

Figure 5. How long did you breastfeed or give pumped breast milk to your baby after delivery?

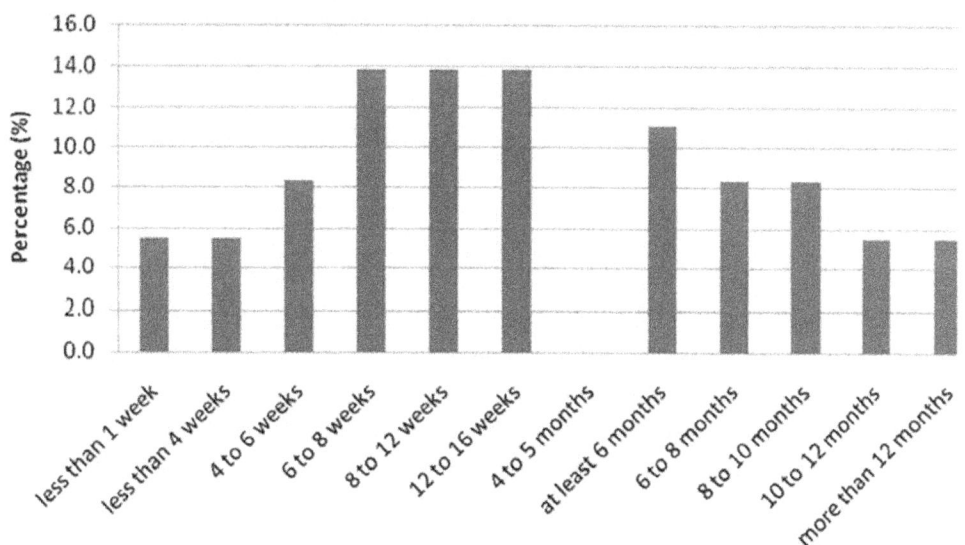

Figure 6. What was the main reason for the stopping of breastfeeding when you did stop?

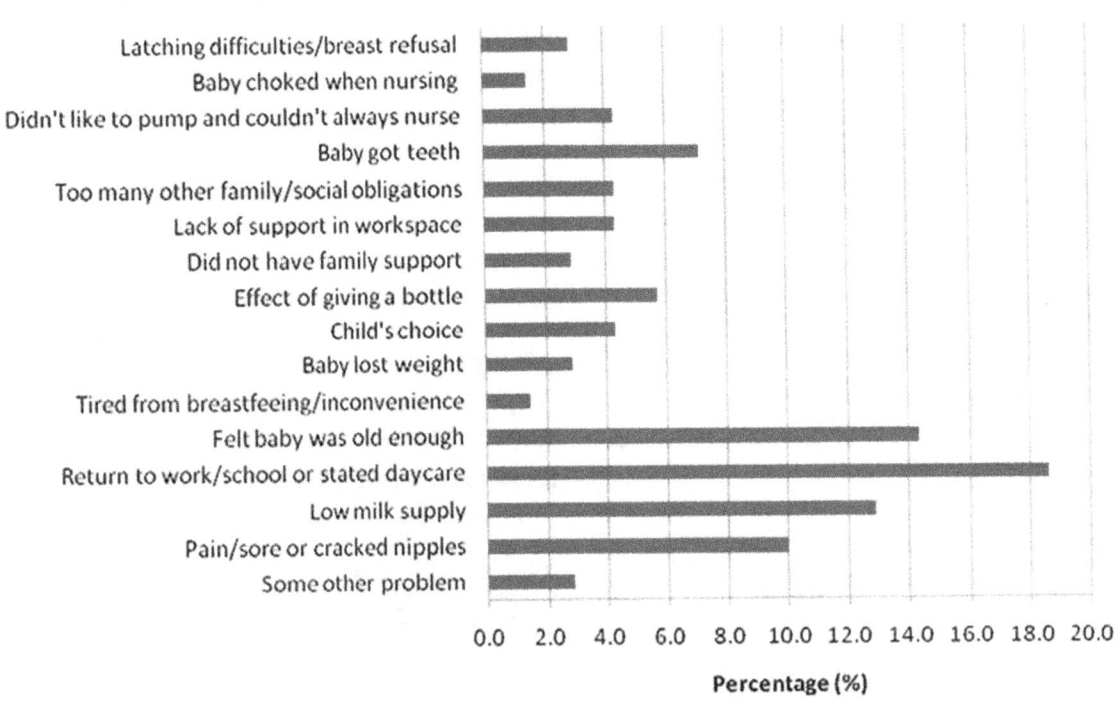

DISCUSSION

Healthy People 2010 objectives for breastfeeding in early postpartum period, at 6 months, and 12 months are 75%, 50%, and 25%, respectively. The national statistics for the United States between the years 1999 and 2005 show that these goals are being approached but have not been reached in actuality (see Table 1). These rates have held fairly steady over the six years, with slight increases each successive year.

Table 1. Percent of U.S. children who were breastfed, by birth year. National Immunization Survey, United States (percent ±half 95% Confidence Interval).

	1999	2000	2001	2002	2003	2004	2005 (provisional)
Early postpartum	68.3±2.9	70.9±1.9	71.6±1.0	71.4±0.9	72.6±0.9	73.1±0.8	74.2±1.2
At 6 months	32.6±2.9	34.2±2.0	36.9±1.2	37.6±1.0	39.1±0.9	42.1±0.9	43.1±1.3
At 12 months	15.0±2.1	15.7±1.5	18.2±0.9	19.0±0.8	19.6±0.8	21.4±0.8	21.4±1.1

Source: http://www.cdc.gov/breastfeeding/data/NIS_data/index.htm

The results from the local survey showed a large number of mothers stopped breastfeeding before 6 months of age. This is probably due to the fact that most of the mothers surveyed went back to work or school by the time their baby was 6 months old. However, some mothers continued to breastfeed, or give breast milk in a bottle, through 12 months.

Table 2. Percent of children who were breastfed in local survey.

	2008
Early postpartum	61.2
At 6 months	11.1
At 12 months	11.2

Healthy People 2010 objectives for exclusive breastfeeding through 3 and 6 months of age are 40% and 17%, respectively. The national statistics for the United States between the years 2003 and 2005 show that these goals are being approached but have not been reached in actuality (see Table 3).

Table 3. Rates of exclusive breastfeeding through 3 and 6 months of age by birth year. National Immunization Survey, United States (percent ±half 95% Confidence Interval).

	2003	2004	2005 (provisional)
Through 3 months	29.6±1.5	31.5±0.9	31.5±1.3

| **Through 6 months** | 10.3±1.0 | 12.1±0.7 | 11.9±0.9 |

Source: http://www.cdc.gov/breastfeeding/data/NIS_data/index.htm

The survey used in the local study did not specify if breastfeeding was exclusive or not. It was observed that in response to the question, "While you were in the hospital or birth center, was your baby fed water, formula, or sugar water at any time?" that several (20) responded that the baby was given these items as supplement to being breastfed. Since, for some babies, this practice may lead to nipple confusion or a decrease in the mother's milk supply, more education should be offered during the prenatal period concerning this practice (The Baby-Friendly Hospital Initiative). In 2007, the CDC conducted the mPINC survey, which reported that newborn feeding practices in 24% of the facilities "reported giving supplements (and not breast milk exclusively) as a general practice with more than half of all healthy, full-term breastfeeding newborns, a practice that is not supportive of breastfeeding" (Centers for Disease Control and Prevention).

Data comparing Louisiana to the United States as a whole are seen in Tables 4, 5, and 6. Louisiana lags behind the national average in breastfeeding, exclusive breastfeeding, and in formula supplementation. In this last area it is actually a good thing that Louisiana falls behind the national average.

Table 4. Provisional Geographic-specific Breastfeeding Rates among Children born in 2005 (Percent +/- half 95% Confidence Interval)

State	Number	Ever Breastfeeding	Breastfeeding at 6 months	Breastfeeding at 12 months
US National	15269	74.2±1.2	43.1±1.3	21.4±1.1
LOUISIANA	302	47.9±7.2	21.8±5.5	9.5±4.1

Source: National Center for Chronic Disease Prevention and Health Promotion

Table 5. Provisional Geographic-specific Exclusive Breastfeeding Rates among Children born in 2005□(Percent +/- half 95% Confidence Interval)

State	Number	Exclusive Breastfeeding through 3 months	Exclusive Breastfeeding through 6 months
US National	15014	31.5±1.3	11.9±0.9
LOUISIANA	300	20.1±5.5	7.2±3.8

Source: National Center for Chronic Disease Prevention and Health Promotion

Table 6. Provisional Geographic-specific Formula Supplementation Rates among Children born in 2005 (Percent +/- half 95% Confidence Interval)

State	Number	Formula Supplementation[1] before 2 days of age	Number	Formula Supplementation[1] before 3 months of age

US National	11654	24.7±1.4	9139	38.3±1.8
LOUISIANA	180	17.9±7.3	126	30.2±10.5

[1]Formula supplementation is defined as supplementation of breast milk with formula (with or without other supplementary liquids or solids) among infants breastfed at the age specified (2 days or 3 months). The denominator for the 2 day or 3 month rate is the number of infants breastfeeding at 2 days or 3 months, respectively. Formula supplementation rates at 6 months are not shown by geographic area due to an insufficient number of women breastfeeding at 6 months in many geographic areas.
Source: National Center for Chronic Disease Prevention and Health Promotion

A map shows a breakdown of the U.S. by states, and Louisiana is in the lowest percentage category for breastfeeding for 6 months, along with six other states. An increase in education about the importance of breastfeeding and how it can benefit both mother and baby is needed in these seven states (see Map 1).

Map 1: Percent of Children Breastfed at 6 Months of Age by State among Children Born in 2005 (Provisional)

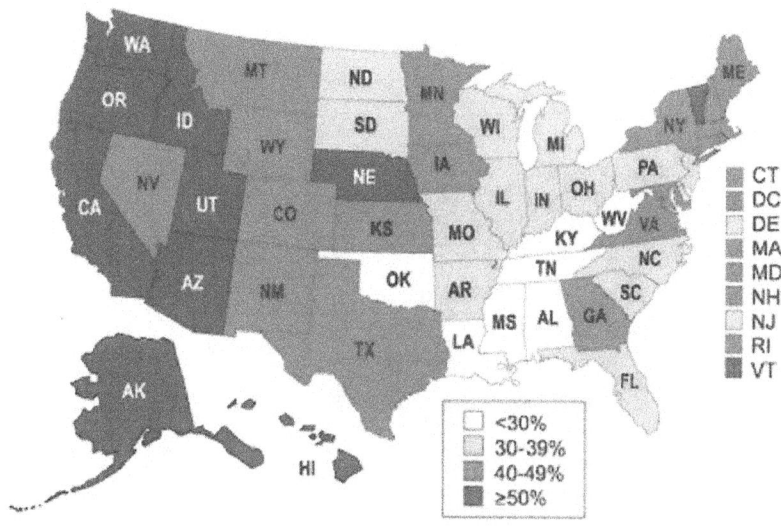

Source: National Immunization Survey, Centers for Disease Control and Prevention, Department of Health and Human Services

In the local survey results, 93.3% of the mothers responding to the survey had education of at least some college on up to Master's degree level. So it is reasonable to say that this is a higher educated population than the average mother in Baton Rouge. According to Cindy Harmon-Jones in *Leaven*, a publication of La Leche League International, "in 2002, on average, breastfeeding mothers in the United States were older, had higher socioeconomic status, and higher education levels than formula feeding mothers" (2005). The results from the local survey agree with this observation. A majority of the respondents were Caucasian, which also could have affected the outcome of the results. It should be pointed out that the researchers attempted to distribute surveys to a more diverse population concerning race, ethnicity, and education levels but circumstances prevented this attempt from succeeding. More research of the local population in Baton Rouge, LA is needed across a more heterogeneous group.

REFERENCES

The Baby-Friendly Hospital Initiative http://www.unicef.orglprogrammelbreastfeedingl baby.htmAccessed January 3, 2009.

Centers for Disease Control and Prevention. Breastfeeding practice-results from the National Immunization Survey.

http://www.cdc. gov /breastfeeding/ dataINIS _ datal2004/socio-demographic.htm Accessed November 22, 2008.

Centers for Disease Control and Prevention. Breastfeeding-Related Maternity Practices at Hospitals and Birth Centers --- United States, 2007.http://www.cdc.gov/mmwr/ preview/mmwrhtml/mm5723al.htm

Accessed January 3, 2009.

Healthy People 2010, U.S. Department of Health and Human Services. *Healthy People 2010.* 2nd ed. Washington, DC: U.S. Department of Health and Human Services; 2000; 46-48.

Harmon-Jones, C. (2005, OctINov). Reading and Evaluating Breastfeeding Research. *Leaven,* 99-103.

La Leche League International. All about La Leche League. http://www.llli.orglab. html?m=1 Accessed November 22, 2008.

Morse, J., & Bottorff, J. (1989, Nov/Dec). Intending to breastfeed and work. JOGNN, 493-500.

U.S. Department of Health and Human Services, Office on Women's Health. Breastfeeding: HHS Blueprint for Action on Breastfeeding. Washington, DC: U.S. Department of Health and Human Services, Office on Women's Health: 2000.

U.s. Preventive Services Task Fore. Behavioral interventions to promote breastfeeding. http://www.ahrq.gov/clinic/3rduspstflbrstfeedlbrfeedrr.htm

Accessed November 22, 2008.

ARTIFICIALLY SWEETENED BEVERAGE CONSUMPTION AND PORTION CONTROL BY AFRICAN AMERICAN FEMALE COLLEGE STUDENTS

By:

Carmela Abels BS
&
Dottie Kenda BS

A research manuscript in Partial fulfillment of the Requirements of the Southern University Dietetic Internship

FOOD AND HUMAN NUTRITION
DIVISION OF FAMILY AND CONSUMER SCIENCES
COLLEGE OF AGRICULTURAL, FAMILY AND CONSUMER SCIENCES
SOUTHERN UNIVERSITY AND A&M COLLEGE

ABSTRACT

Objective
To determine if an association exists between the consumption of beverages artificially sweetened with sugar substitutes (intense sweeteners, nonnutritive sweeteners, or artificial sweeteners) and the control of food portions in managing caloric intake among African American female college students.

Design
A cross-sectional questionnaire was used to collect data.

Participants/Setting
A convenience sample of 50 African American female college students (mean age=20 years; mean Body Mass Index = 27) who consumed artificially sweetened beverages were recruited from a Baton Rouge, Louisiana university campus.

Statistical analyses
Both descriptive statistics and statistical analyses were used (data were summarized in percentages or mean ±standard deviation). Relationships between attitudes regarding eating habits were calculated using Spearman correlation coefficients. Relationships between Body Mass Index (BMI), portion control, and number of artificially sweetened beverages consumed per day were calculated using Pearson correlation coefficients.

Results
There was no significant correlation between portion control and the consumption of artificially sweetened beverages ($r=0.076$; $P<0.05$). Additionally, there was no statistically significant correlation between BMI and portion control ($r=-0.129$; $P<0.05$). A weak, direct correlation was found between BMI ($r=0.308$; $P<0.05$) and the consumption of artificially sweetened beverages. However, a significant positive correlation ($r=0.391$; $P<0.01$) was observed between participants who reported consuming medium-sized fast food meal products. Twenty-five percent of the participants who consumed the large-sized fast food meals were obese and nine percent of the participants were normal weight based on BMI calculations.

Conclusions
There are few studies exploring the relationship between the consumption of nonnutritive sweetened beverages and portion control as a possible approach to the overweight and obesity problem, specifically in college females. This study did not show a correlation between portion control and the consumption of artificially sweetened beverages. A full exploration of this association requires additional information about use patterns of non-nutritive sweeteners, examination of information concerning the whole diet and patterns of energy expenditure, and preferably, long-term randomized, controlled trials in larger populations.

INTRODUCTION

Does artificially sweetened beverage consumption help with weight maintenance or lead to overconsumption of energy dense food? There has been a great deal of research over the last twenty years resulting in contradicting evidence in an attempt to answer the sugar-substitute (nonnutritive sweeteners, intense sweeteners, artificial sweeteners) and over-consumption correlation. The debate continues whether intense sweeteners increase appetite for sweet foods, promote overeating, and lead to weight gain or have little to no effect.

Interpreting the association between sugar sweetened (nutritive) beverage consumption and nutrient intake is complex, but a review of studies shows a link between soft drink intake and increased energy consumption. From 1977-2001, calorie intake from soft drinks and fruit drinks increased by 135% and the prevalence of adult obesity increased by 200%. Consumption of sugar-sweetened beverages (SSB's) has been associated with the obesity epidemic and type 2 diabetes. Research has shown that successful weight management, however, requires a conscious control of energy intake, healthy lifestyle, and maintenance of a low-energy diet. Context and dietary behavior then become more pertinent to energy intake than a physiologic satiety deficit after liquid sugar consumption.

Body weight will increase if energy intake is greater than energy expenditure. In an effort to decrease energy intake and maintain or lose weight, some individuals use artificial sweeteners instead of sugar. A zero energy diet drink that replaces an energy-containing food should result in less stored energy (adipose tissue). Current research has shown, however, that the body can adjust to the decreased intake of energy associated with the use of artificial sweetener. One mechanism could be that NNSs activate taste reward circuits but may not fully satisfy a desire for natural caloric sweet ingestion and the individual seeks out calories, thereby defeating the use of NNS drinks. In addition, the use of nonnutritive sweetened drinks could lead consumers to change their eating behavior and actually increase energy intake. This could occur if the expected energy savings from the artificially sweetened drink is greater than any actual, rationalized caloric overconsumption. Research evidence suggests that is nonnutritive sweeteners (NNS) are used as substitutes for higher energy yielding sweeteners, they can help with weight management, but whether they will be used in this way is uncertain. This will require additional information about use patterns of NNS, clarification of information concerning the entire diet and patterns of energy expenditure and long-term randomized, controlled trials I free-living populations.

In the United States, approximately 15 million adolescents and young adults are enrolled in college with 35% being overweight or obese. There are no studies exploring the relationship between the consumption of nonnutritive sweeteners and portion control as a possible approach to overweight and obesity problem, specifically in college females.

Does a relationship exist between the consumption of beverages sweetened with sugar substitutes (intense sweeteners, nonnutritive sweeteners, or artificial sweeteners) and the control of food portions in managing caloric intake among female college students? This question arises from the paucity of information surrounding diet beverage consumption and dietary habits of college females. The questions put forth in this study will attempt to generate a hypothesis on the relationship between NNS beverages and portion control by college females.

In conclusion, consumption of sugar-sweetened beverages has been associated with the obesity epidemic and type 2 diabetes. Sweeteners add to food palatability and dieting patterns consisting of foods of low palatability have shown inconsistent, limited success. One method of reducing caloric intake has been to substitute artificial sweeteners for nutritive sweeteners in food and beverages. Approximately 15% of the U.S. Population uses artificial sweeteners, and the number is rising. There has been a great deal of research over the last twenty years resulting in contradicting evidence in an attempt to answer the sugar-substitute, (nonnutritive sweeteners, intense sweeteners, artificial sweeteners) and over-consumption correlation. The debate continues whether sugar substitutes by themselves increase appetite for sweet foods, promote overeating, and lead to weight gain, or have little or no effect on dietary intake. A recent perspective has determined that artificial sweeteners offer no benefits for weight loss or weight maintenance without energy restriction. Research has shown that successful weight management requires a conscious control of energy intake, a healthy lifestyle, and maintenance of a low-energy diet.

This study addresses the lack of evidence on the concomitant consumption of artificially sweetened beverages and portion control as an influence on weight maintenance or weight gain by trying to determine whether a relationship exists between the two practices. The working hypothesis was that there would be no significant positive correlation between the consumption of artificially sweetened beverages and portion control among this population.

GOAL & OBJECTIVES

The objective of this study is to describe (define, quantify?) the relationship between artificially sweetened (intensely sweetened, nonnutritive sweetened) beverage consumption and control of food portions in managing caloric intake in a select population (African American college females).

METHODS

(PARTICIPANTS AND METHODS)
Study Population and Eligibility Criteria

A convenience sample of female college students' age 18-35 years were approached by dietetic interns at the colleges' student union or eating facility. The participants were recruited from Southern University located in Baton Rouge, Louisiana. During their lunch hour, they were offered an opportunity to volunteer for an anonymous survey. Potential participants responded to the interns in person and completed preliminary eligibility screening, which included confirmation that the potential participant was enrolled at the university, claimed artificially sweetened (diet) drinks were their beverage of choice, and would be willing to answer a survey. Exclusion criteria were those who were unwilling to give informed consent and those female college students who did not consumer diet soft drinks.

Survey Instrument

The 24-question survey instrument was developed specifically for this study. The survey Included demographic items (age, education, and race), anthropometric information (height and weight), attitudes relating to eating habits and portion control, and asked about consumption of artificially sweetened beverages. Students were asked how often they had consumed artificially sweetened beverages in a day (Table 1). Frequency categories for beverages consumption for any type of artificially sweetened 9diet) beverages ranged from "one" to "more than four per day".

Perception to eating habits and portion control was also assessed. Students were asked to endorse the statement that best described their current calorie intake. Students were also asked to rate their eating habits and their knowledge of food portion sizes on the survey; four categories ranged from "poor to excellent". Perceived number of calories consumed per day was assessed; five categories ranged from "much too low" to much too high. Perceived familiarity with portion control to maintain or aid in losing weight and perceived likeability to follow a diet that includes portion control was assessed; four categories ranged from "not at all" to "very".

The survey was also used to assess behaviors relating to the portion size consumption. The students were asked to report the frequency of fast-food intake on the survey; five categories ranged from "one to more than 4" times a week. Subsequently, the portion size of fast-food intake was asked; four categories ranged from "small" to "supersize".

Age, student status, race, height, and weight were self-reported on the survey. Weight status categories were defined according to current body mass index (BMI; calculated as kg/m^2) guidelines for adults (not overweight: BMI<25.0, overweight; BMI = 25.0-29.9, and obese: BMI≥BMI 30.0).

Statistical Analysis

The dependent variable of this study was BMI. Descriptive statistics were computed for the characteristics of the participants (mean and standard deviation) and to examine differences in attitudes relating to eating habits and portion control of female college students. Relationships between attitudes relating to eating habits and portion control were explored using Spearman's correlation coefficients. Pearson correlation coefficients were used to test for associations between BMI, number of artificially sweetened beverages, and portion control. Data were analyzed using the Statistical Package for Social Sciences (version 12.0.1, 2003, SPSS Inc., Chicago, IL) software, and the results were determined to be significant if the P value was less than the critical value of 0.05. Data were summarized in percentages of as the mean ± standard deviation.

RESULTS
Participant Characteristics

Sixty-three college students volunteered for and participated in the study (100% female and 100% African American). Students were excluded from the analyses if they did not complete the survey (n=1), or they did not consume artificially sweetened beverages (n=12). These exclusions resulted in a final sample number for analyses of 50 students. The sample ranged across all grade levels, with the sample composed of 22% freshman, 48% sophomores, 8% juniors, 20% seniors, and 2% graduate students. The majority of the students were under the age of 22, with the range of 18-to 35 years. Mean age and BMI for African-American female college students was 20 years and 29 respectively.

Description and Correlation of Participant's Attitudes Regarding their Eating Habits

The majority of the participants agreed their eating habits were fair (60%) and their knowledge of food portion sizes were fair (42%) or good (42%). Although, most of the participants indicated they are familiar with controlling portion sizes to maintain or aid in losing consumed per day were somewhat high, and if they were on a diet that includes portion control, they would somewhat (36%) or fairly (36%) be likely to follow one (Table 2).

Attitudes regarding personal eating habits showed a weak, direct correlation (r=0.341; P<0.05) with perceived knowledge of food portion sizes, and a weak, inverse correlation with their perceived number of calories consumed per day. The perceived likeability to follow a diet that includes portion control showed a weak, inverse correlation (r=0.121; P<0.05) with their eating habits, and a significant (r=0.391; P<0.01) with perceived familiarity with portion control and weight maintenance or loss (Table 3). Approximately 38% of the participants indicated they control their food portions at each eating occasion.

Interpretations of BMI and Portion Size

Characteristics of the study population are presented in Table 4. Results indicate the majority (68%) of the participants in the normal (mean [M] = 21.8, standard deviation = 1.6), overweight [M] = 27.7, standard deviation = 1.5), and obese (mean [M] = 24.5 standard deviation = 6.2) group ordered the medium-sized meals when consuming fast food products. When comparing the consumption of large-sized meals, 25% of the participants were obese and 9% were of normal weight.

Correlations of BMI, Portion Size and Beverage Intake

BMI showed a weak, direct correlation (r=0.308); P<0.05) with the consumption of artificially sweetened beverages (See Table 5). Thus, as BMI mean increased, the number of artificially sweetened beverages per day increased (See Figure). Thirty-two percent indicated they drink artificially sweetened beverages to maintain their weight and 28% indicated they drink the beverages to lose weight. There were no statistically significant correlations between BMI and portion control (r=0.129; P<0.05) (See Table 5).

Graphs and Tables follow in the appendix.

DISCUSSION

The study showed no significant correlation between the consumption of artificially sweetened beverages and dietary portion control. The study did, however, confirm previous research findings that show the co-existence of increased BMI and consumption of artificially sweetened beverages. This finding does not indicate that a correlation exists, only that the two exist together.

Information for the study was obtained from personal interviews conducted using a written questionnaire. The participants were asked to individually fill out the questionnaire, but could ask for question clarification from the researcher. In this way, response rates were higher, responses could be probed, and participants could clarify their answers. This method of collecting information was an advantage over questionnaires completed at a remote location and returned by mail and was considered a strength.

A limitation of this study was that this survey instrument was not validated even though it was based upon questionnaires used in similar studies. In addition, the cross sectional data could not provide a long term perspective. The small number of participants aided the interview process, but precluded providing robust data. Findings were specific to this particular population and not generalizable. Even with these limitations, findings from this study showed no deviation from a January 2009 comprehensive review of studies done on nonnutritive sweeteners and appetite and food intake. Findings from previous studies revealed:

- There is no proof that artificial sweeteners added to non-energy-yielding products increase appetite
- Evidence of long-term success of substitution of artificial sweeteners for nutritive sweeteners for weight management is not available.
- The addition of artificial sweeteners to diets is not beneficial for weight loss or reduced weight gain without energy restriction

CONCLUSION

Based upon study results, the date were not strong enough to reject the hypothesis that there would be no significant positive correlation between the consumption of artificially sweetened beverages and portion control among the study participants. The study did focus on a health issue that has not been well investigated to date. One avenue for further research would be to stud the amount and direction (positive or negative) of influence these sweeteners have on the ability to moderate energy intakes by controlling portion amounts. In total, the data point to the need for further study and suggest that artificially sweetened beverage consumption and portion control could influence weight issues among female college students.

APPENDICES

APPENDIX
Graphs:

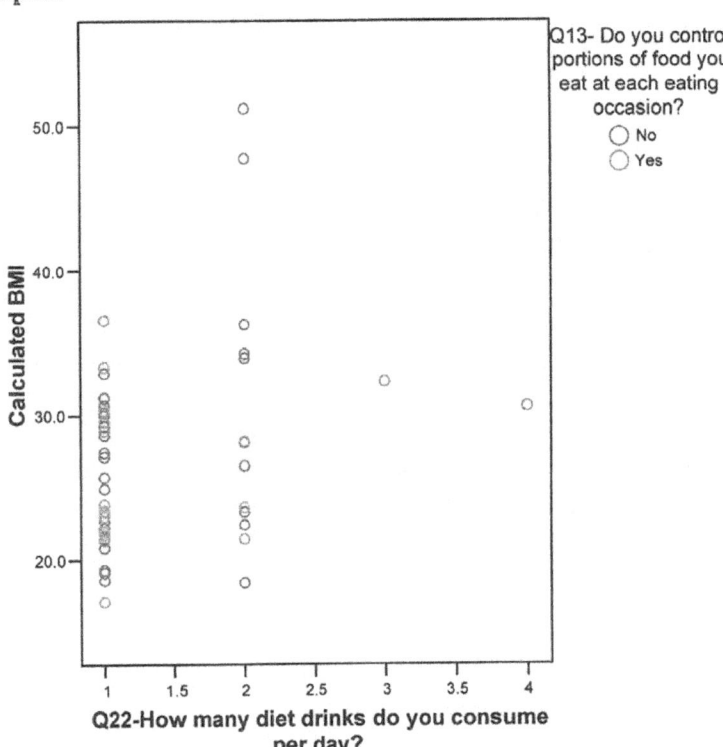

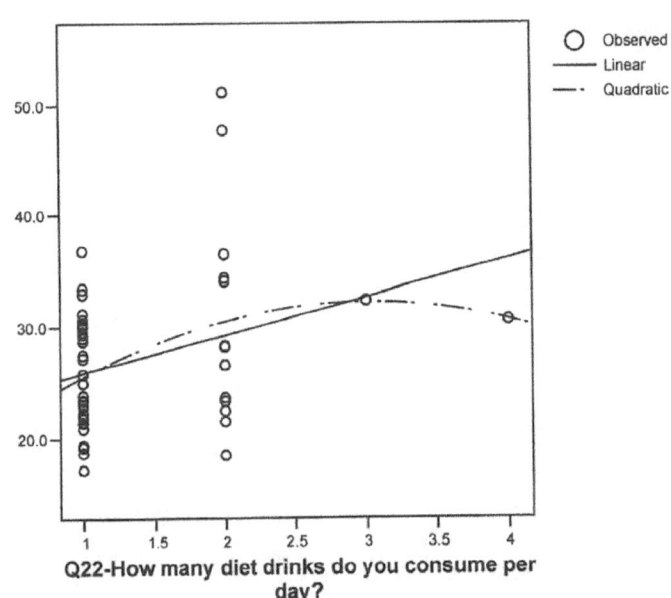

Calculated BMI

Tables:

Table 1. Sample Survey items
Demographic Information
1. Age
2. Education Level_____ Year in College
3. Race: (check one)____African American ____Hispanic ____White (Non-Hispanic) ____Other
Anthropometric Information
1.Current weight:____
2. Height: ____
Eating Habits:

1. How would you rate your eating habits?
   1. Poor
   2. Fair
   3. Good
   4. Excellent

2. For someone of your age, height, and weight, do you feel that the number of calories you eat per day is?
   1. Much Too Low
   2. Somewhat Low
   3. Just About Right
   4. Somewhat High
   5. Much Too High

3. Do you control the portions of food you eat at each eating occasion?
   0. No
   1. Yes

4. How many times per week do you dine out or consume "fast food"?
   1. 1
   2. 2
   3. 3
   4. 4
   5. More than 4

5. When consuming "fast food products" which size meal do you usually order?
   1. Small
   2. Medium
   3. Large
   4. Supersize

6. How would you rate your knowledge of food portion sizes?
    1. Poor
    2. Fair
    3. Good
    4. Excellent

7. Do you consume artificially sweetened (diet) drinks?
    0. No
    1. Yes

8. How many artificially sweetened drinks do you consume per day?
    1. 1
    2. 2
    3. 3
    4. 4
    5. More than 4

9. How familiar are you with portion control to maintain or aid in losing weight?
    1. Not at all
    2. Somewhat Low
    3. Fairly
    4. Very

10. How likely are you to follow a diet that includes portion control?
    1. Not at all
    2. Somewhat Low
    3. Fairly
    4. Very

Table 2. Comparisons for attitudes relating to eating habits and portion control among female college student participants[a]

	Poor	Fair		Good	Excellent	
	←		% (n)		→	
Attitudes regarding eating habits						
Perceived eating habits	16.0 (8)	60.0 (30)		22.0 (11)	2.0 (1)	
Perceived knowledge of food portion sizes	10.0 (5)	42.0 (21)		42.0 (21)	6.0 (3)	

	Much too low	Somewhat low		Just about right	Somewhat high	Much too high
	←		% (n)		→	
Attitudes regarding eating habits						
Perceived number of calories consumed per day	4.0 (2)	6.0 (3)		30.0 (15)	52.0 (26)	8.0 (4)

	Not at all	Somewhat		Fairly	Very	
	←		% (n)		→	
Attitudes regarding eating habits						
Perceived familiarity with portion control and weight maintenance or weight loss	20.0 (10)	44.0 (22)		22.0 (11)	14.0 (7)	
Perceived likeability to follow a diet that includes portion control	8.0 (4)	36.0 (18)		36.0 (18)	20.0 (10)	

[a] Unadjusted percentages, weighted to reflect the probability of responding to the survey.

Table 3. Correlation coefficients for attitudes relating to eating habits and portion control among female college student participants[a]					
	Perceived eating habits	Perceived knowledge of food portion sizes	Perceived number of calories consumed per day	Perceived familiarity with portion control and weight maintenance or loss	Perceived ability to follow a diet that includes portion control
Attitudes regarding eating habits					
Perceived eating habits	1.00				
Perceived knowledge of food portion sizes	.341*	1.00			
Perceived number of calories consumed per day	-.327*	-.194	1.00		
Perceived familiarity with portion control and weight maintenance or loss	.035	0.179	-.024	1.00	
Perceived likeability to follow a diet that includes portion control	-.121*	0.169	0.153	.391**	1.00
[a] Unadjusted and unweighted Spearman's correlation coefficients * P < 0.05 ** P < 0.01					

Table 4. Results from multivariate regression analysis of data collected from female college student participants that evaluate the association between dietary practices and BMI

Dependent variable	Parameter	$\beta \pm$Standard error
BMI	Intercept	
	Component 1: The practice of portion control during eating occasion	-.154±2.280
	Component 2: The number of diet soft drinks consumed per day	.320±1.480

Table 4A. Age and anthropometric characteristics of underweight (UW),normal-weight (NW), overweight (OW), and obese (O) participants who surveyed to consuming small, medium, large, supersize portions when eating "fast food products

Varia-bles	Small Portion			Medium Portion			Large Portion			Supersize Portion		
	NW	OW	O	NW	OW	O	NW	OW	O	NW	OW	O
	n=22	n=11	n=16	n=22	n=11	n=16	n=22	n=11	n=16	n=22	n=11	n=16
	mean ± standard deviation											
Age	25.3±6.5	19.0±.0	21.0±2.0	19.8±1.3	20.6±4.1	19.8±1.3	19.0±0.0	0.0±0	19.3±1.9	0.0±0.0	0.0±0.0	27.0±0.0
Height (in)	64.3±2.9	59.0±.0	63.7±4.0	65.3±2.5	63.1±3.8	64.4±3.1	64.0±4.2	0.0±0	64.5±1.7	0.0±0.0	0.0±0.0	60.0±0.0
Weight (lb)	130.0±14.5	111.0±0.0	178.7±0.0	131.8±14.1	161.6±15.2	201.5±35.2	126.5±17.7	0.0±0	223.5±44.5	0.0±0.0	0.0±0.0	175.0±0.0
BMI[a]	22.5±2.3	29.0±.0	30.9±0.5	21.7±1.6	27.6±1.5	34.2±5.9	21.7±0.2	0.0±0	38.0±9.1	0.0±0.0	0.0±0.0	34.2±0.0

[a]BMI = body mass index; calculated kg/m²

Table 5. Pearson correlation coefficients for associations between BMI, portion control, and number of artificially sweetened beverage consumption among female college participants.

	BMI	Portion Control	Number of Artificially Sweetened Beverages
BMI	1.00		
Portion Control	-0.129	1.00	
Number of artificially sweetened beverages	.308*	0.076	1.00
* P < 0.05.			

Figures:

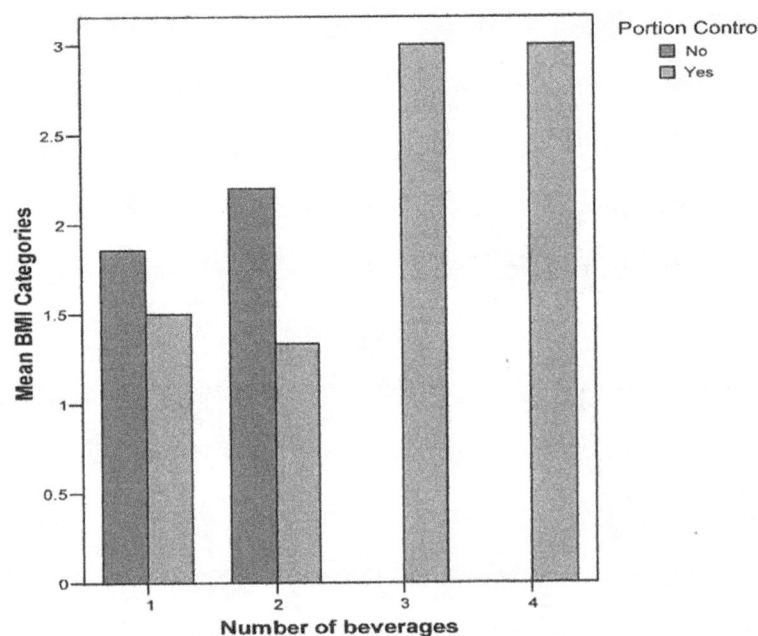

Figure 1. Relationship between the Mean BMI categories (underweight, normal weight, overweight, and obese) (scale 0-3) and the number of artificially sweetened beverages consumed per day in African-American female college students who indicated that they either do or do not practice portion control during each eating occasion.

REFERENCES

Benton D. Can artificial sweeteners help control body weight and prevent obesity? Nutr Research Reviews. 2005; 18:63-76.

Mattes RD, Popkin BM. Nonnutritive sweetener consumption in humans: effects on appetite and food intake and their putative mechanisms. *Am J Clin Nutr.* 2009; 89: 1-14.

Bellisle F, Drewnowski A. Intense sweeteners, energy intake and the control of body weight. *EJCN* 2007; 61: 691-700.

Drewnowski A, Bellisle F. Liquid calories, sugar, and body weight. *AmJClinNutr. 2007; 85:651*-61.

Bleich SN, Wang YC, Wang Y, Gortmaker SL. Increasing consumption of sugar-sweetened beverages among US adults: 1988-1994 to 1999-2004. *Am J Clin Nutr. 2009; 89:372-81.*

Malik VS, Schulze MB, Hu FB. Intake of sugar-sweetened beverages and weight gain: a systematic review. *Am J Clin Nutr. 2006; 84:274-88.*

Vartanian LR, Schwartz MB, Brownell KD. Effects of soft drink consumption on nutrition and health: a systematic review and meta-analysis. *AJPH.* 2007:97(4): 667-675.

Frank GKW, Obemdorfer TA, Simmons AN, Paulus MP, Fudge JL, Yang TT, Kayeb WHo Sucrose activates human taste pathways differently from artificial sweetener. *Neurolmage.2008; 39:1559-1569.*

Huffman L, West DS. Readiness to change sugar sweetened beverage intake among college students. *EatBeh. 2007; 8(1):10-14.*

Cluskey M, Grobe D. College weight gain and behavior transitions: male and female differences. *JADA.2009; 109(2):325-329.*

Bowman SA. Beverage choices of young females: changes and impact on nutrient intakes. *JADA. 2002; 102:1234-1239.*

West DS, Bursae Z, Quimby D, Prewitt TE, Spatz T, Nash C, Mays G, Eddings K. Self-reported sugar-sweetened beverage intake among college students. *Obesity.* 2006; 14: 1825-1831.